FLIGHT MEDICINE: The Pursuit of Excellence

Dan Turner

FOREWARD

A simple Google search for " mentor' reveals vernaculars such as "an experienced expert," "a well educated trainer", and "an individual who teaches a less experienced person". Well, I'll need to write Miriam-Webster and let them know this term is falling short. Dan Turner far exceeds and surpasses these definitions.

I worked incredibly hard to earn the privilege of wearing a flight suit for AirCare with the University of Mississippi Medical Center. Once there, I realized the flight suit was only a false peak, and I had a lot more climbing to do to get to the true summit of being a competent and skillful clinician. At that time I was hired, and undoubtedly still, there were some highly accomplished clinicians, and Dan was one of the few on top.

To earn Dan's respect and trust, you would need to be magnanimous and approaching the limits of perfection. It is one reason, I assume, why Donna Norris, chief flight nurse and program director, choose him to train the incoming orientees, because once you earned Dan's approval, you actually were a well-trained, and competent critical care transport clinician. I began my training looking forward to working with all the transport greats, and on my first shift with him, I knew he would be tough to impress. Fortunately, Dan is kind and tender to the neophyte transport clinician, and additionally has an amazing ability to bring humor into training moments. You would feel comfortable with receiving the scrutiny that has to come with critical care transport training. You'd laugh, which would loosen you up, and then you'd be more welcoming to any professional criticism offered. I learned so much with him and am so grateful to have had that opportunity. I have learned a lot of emergency and critical care medicine in my career, and can honestly say that I have never learned more than my years at AirCare where I was highly influenced by Dan Turner.

I remember the day I received the news about Dan's accident. I cried. I knew the world was about to lose one of the greatest people and clinicians ever to grace the world. Then, without surprise, Dan rose from the ashes created by the accident, finished his schooling, continued to inspire others, and now has written this concise work that is worth more than a thousand volumes of medical texts and hundreds of hours of training. This book is simply the figurehead of the unfinished legacy of Dan Turner. As an educator, author, flight paramedic, and athlete, I know that this book will influence you to challenge your own limits, inspire you to be greater, and dare you to change the world.

Dan, thank you for advice, guidance, and friendship. Most importantly, thank you for redefining the term 'mentorship'. In doing so, you have truly impacted your patient's, colleagues, and countless strangers.

Charles F. Swearingen, BS, NRP, FP-C
Owner, Meducation Specialists
National Athlete, USA Volleyball
Colleague, Friend, and Fan of Dan "The Man" Turner.

[Intentionally left blank]

ACKNOWLEDGMENTS

I only wish to thank one person: Charlie Swearingen. Thanks for helping me when I really needed

[Intentionally Left Blank]

CHAPTER 1: HOW IT ALL STARTED

I was 20 years old, working as an electrician's apprentice. At the time, I was helping to run conduit and pull wire at a renovation at Southwest Mississippi Regional Medical Center in McComb, MS. There I was, in the early Mississippi summer, working in hot blue jeans and uncomfortable work boots. Every now and then, I'd see hospital personnel walk outside in their comfortable-looking scrubs and tennis shoes and I got to thinking, "Man, I want that"! I also had a good friend, Joe Nettles, who had finished nursing school, quickly secured a new job, and was able to buy a brand new car. Together, the aforementioned observations were enough to motivate me to embark on the greatest career that I ever could have imagined. I realized that first, I had to go back to school. I also realized that I needed a job-schedule that would allow me to go back to school. I spoke with the chief nursing officer and there just so happened to have an upcoming ECG course that the hospital used to train people as cardiac monitor technicians for the hospital's telemetry floor. The course lasted one week and I found myself really enjoying the subject material and I passed the test at the end of the week. I was hired as an ECG monitor tech and finally had an evening job that would allow me to go to school during the day and best of all, I was able to wear comfortable scrubs and tennis shoes to work—I had arrived. One evening, while working one evening after school, I remember hearing a thunderous sound outside and one of my co-workers was standing at a window and said, "Dan, quick—come here"! I peeked at my 30 ECG readings to make sure everyone looked alright and then hurried to the window to see what was going on. To my total surprise, I saw a helicopter landing on the hospital helipad. Like a little kid, I was totally thrilled with what I saw. I asked my coworker, "who is that"? She explained that the people disembarking from the aircraft were a nurse and paramedic from Jackson, MS. I was totally blown away and I decided at that moment, that I was going to do that one day—no doubt in my mind.

Nursing school was the hardest thing I'd ever been through. Suddenly, I found myself in a "foreign land," learning a "foreign language," and learning about physiological processes that I never learned in high school Biology class. After graduation, I worked for a year as a RN on that same telemetry floor until getting my first ER job in Brookhaven, MS at King's Daughters Medical Center (KDMC). I was lucky enough to have a super-cool boss, Jane Jones, that encouraged continuing education and obtaining certifications that showed proficiency in my chosen emergency medicine specialty. It was there, in that emergency department that I really started to grow as a critical care/emergency nurse. I will always be grateful to Mrs. Jane for shaping me into the nurse that I became. It was also at KDMC that I gained an appreciation and respect for paramedics. See, KDMC has their own ambulance service and when the medics were in between their calls, they would walk over to the ER to help and hang out. The ones that I especially remember making an impression on me are:

Jimmy Martin, Sandra McDavid Martin, Ricky Alford, Kim Nelson, Lonnie Ferrell, John Hart, and Bert Cline. I always thought it was cool how they always seemed ready for anything and had the cool gear stowed away in their cargo pockets and belts (i.e. scissors, folding knives with glass-breakers, etc.). Not only were they true professionals, they were super people to visit with and learn from. I'll never forget them, even after all of these years. It was then that my in-hospital experiences converged with the pre-hospital experiences of others.

CHAPTER 2: MY NEXT STEPS

In that emergency department in Brookhaven, I had a good variety of experiences. I helped my colleagues treat gunshot wounds, stabbings, heart attacks, and high-speed motor vehicle crashes from the nearby interstate. I learned defibrillation and transcutaneous pacing for slow heart rates. I would have to say, the best learning experiences that I had in that emergency department was the ability to talk to the ER doctors and ask questions, like: why did you order that test and what is that test going to tell us? I would say that experience was invaluable in giving me confidence and the ability to think for myself in the years to come.

My next step was to find out where I needed to go to find a helicopter team. It took some asking around and a few phone calls, but I learned of the University of Mississippi Medical Center's (UMMC) AirCare team was a good place to check. I called into their office and setup an appointment to meet and talk with the flight crew on duty. A couple of weeks went by and it was finally time to go talk to the 2-man crew on duty. These were the two medical crew members— not the pilot.

After I arrived and met up with Flight Nurse Bo Sullivan and Flight Paramedic Mike Ellis. They were on their way to check equipment and gear in the aircraft—how exciting! When we made it to the aircraft, I was awe-struck by that flying machine that had been customized to transport and treat one patient at a time. The site was truly amazing to me.

Inside the aircraft, there were many zippered packs and other equipment placed in a particular way, so it could be reached quickly when needed. I thought that was very cool. We spent several minutes discussing medications they frequently used and that they didn't work based on specific doctor's orders. Instead, they worked off of protocols written and approved by the team's medical director—which was an ER physician there at the University of Mississippi Medical Center. At this point I was starting to feel a little intimidated. But I also learned that I would need two years of ER and/or ICU experience. We finished up at the aircraft and I departed for home, about 1 ½ hours away.

On the way home I did some quick math and realized I only needed about 6 more months of ER experience before I would even be considered. So I figured that it would be better for me to begin working in the UMMC Adult ER. So, on December 14, 1998, I started orientation at UMMC's Adult ER. The energy in that place was exhilarating. As luck would have it, 7 months after starting at UMMC, there was a position opening up for a flight nurse with AirCare—wow! I put my application in and received a call scheduling an interview. I was so excited, yet scared to death.

The day of the interview arrived and I was very nervous. The interview felt like I was under subpoena for a congressional hearing. I walked in after they called my name and there they were: two medical directors, flight team' chief flight nurse, lead paramedic, and the program manager—all sitting on one side of a table. On the opposite side of the table was a single empty chair—for me! I made it through the interview somehow and departed for a friend's house about 30 minutes away. I spent the afternoon there at my friend's, Mark Randall's house. While there, I received a call from the chief flight nurse, she said, "Hey, this is Donna with AirCare. You wanna come work for me"? I have no idea what I said, but it amounted to an emphatic "YES"!

After starting, I quickly learned that there was more to being on a flight team than just memorizing protocols and medications. Establishing relationships in the community was just as important.

CHAPTER 3: PROFESSIONALISM AND BUILDING RELATIONSHIPS IN THE COMMUNITY

What is your idea of what a flight team member (FTM) should be?

Is it the cool-looking flight suit and boots? Is it the professionalism and friendliness on display when you've encountered a FTM in the past? Maybe it's that no matter the scenario , the FTM confidently takes control and improves the worst of situations. Hopefully, your answer is "all of the above ". A lot will be expected of you by both, your team and your referring agencies. Whatever your idea of what a FTM is, strive everyday to live it. This will contribute greatly to your success.

What do you get when you put a flight suit on a jerk?

A jerk in a flight suit, of course. No one likes an arrogant jerk. Especially when things have gone sideways and a referring agency calls for your help. When I started flying in 1999, I learned very quickly that referring agencies had been insulted by the way they were talked to by a FTM. Sadly, in some cases, FTMs are anticipated to be condescending and arrogant. From very early on in my career, I vowed to change that impression that referring agencies had of FTMs. I not only wanted to be good clinically, I wanted to do it with a

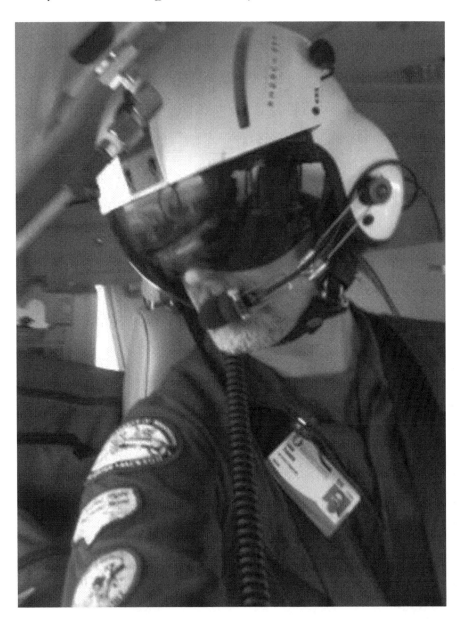

smile on my face. You have to remember, the medical

equipment and your training will be more advanced than some of that of the referring agencies you will serve. Regardless, they've worked hard before you landed with the resources available to them and they always deserve to hear, "good job ". Use hairy situations as an opportunity to teach. Simply explain what needs to be done, explain how you are doing it, and provide feedback on a patient's condition-change. Folks appreciate being a part of a solution. Make friends out there. I promise they'll call you back again and again.

Scope of Practice

This section will be the longest of this chapter because I think it's important for you to know that some days you'll have to make tough decisions and no matter how valiant your motives are, you can step over red lines and risk losing your license. You can be morally and ethically right, but wrong in a legal sense. I'll explain.

Background: each year, in July, when our medical center's new emergency department residents began their residency, we would have a training day in the cadaver lab to learn and practice various life-saving procedures. One that we were taught, in case we were in a situation where there wasn't a capable physician available, was the insertion of a chest tube. For those not familiar with medical jargon, inserting a chest tube is the procedure performed for a patient with a collapsed lung. Little did I know that I'd be in that very situation only 3 years into my 13 1/2-year career.

We were dispatched to a rural hospital on a flight for a 50 year-old obese female with severe shortness of breath. When we arrived, the patient was not in the emergency department, but in radiology, having a CT of her chest performed. As we waited in the room and readied our gear, we heard an excited voice and a fast-moving stretcher coming down the hall toward us. "She's got a tension pneumo"!, we heard a female voice profess. When they arrived into the room, we observed an obese woman, in her 50s, that had labored respirations, no cyanosis, but could not say her name due to dyspnea. The ER doctor was in the room by this time and I noticed he had one arm in a sling. I tried two needle thoracostomies, but the woman's obesity provided a thicker tissue barrier than our angiocatheters could traverse. At this time, needle thoracostomies, or needle decompressions were within my scope of practice—inserting chest tubes was not. I started thinking, we have a 20-minute transport time, she's already short of breath, has a tension pneumothorax confirmed on CT, and needs to be stabilized with a chest tube before we leave with her. I told the doctor, "We need a chest tube doc". He looked down at his arm in a sling and said, "I can't put in a chest tube ". I thought to myself, "Okay, this is why I've had cadaver lab training, one day, for the past 3 years. Since I was going to have to deviate from normal protocol, I called my medical control physician, explained the situation, and told him I was about to put in a chest tube. He agreed and we hung up the phone. I asked for a chest tube tray and the ER staff had it available quickly. I made my initial incision over the fifth intercostal space at the mid-axillary line. Then I punched through the pleura with a pair of curved Kelley forceps. I heard a large rush of air, indicating that the tension was relieved. The patient began to breathe easier. Now it was time to insert the chest tube, suture it in place, and connect the water-seal to suction. All of that was done and I covered the insertion site with a 4x4 gauze and tape. While securing everything, my partner was preparing the aircraft stretcher for moving the patient over. Her vital signs were stable and she was breathing much easier—job well done and I was proud to have had the cadaver lab training. I saved a lady's life today—wow! We completed the transport without incident and I explained what happened to my director and manager. We thought the best thing to do was to self-report the incident to the Board of Nursing. We thought that surely, they'd understand. Boy, were we wrong. What began was a month-long investigation and a few weeks of administrative leave with pay. It was torturous to be off and wondering if I was going to lose my license and career that I had worked so hard for. Well, I didn't lose my license and career, but I did get a letter in my Board file stating I performed duties beyond my scope of practice. I felt it was unfair and when I use the "mama rule", if it was my mama that needed a chest tube and I was the only hope of her getting one, I'd do it all over again. What I want for you to remember is some scenarios you'll find yourself in will be in shades of gray, but the rules that govern you are in black and white. I hope none of you ever find yourself in that position.

Don't be a complainer.

Your colleagues won't like it and your boss will like it even less. Instead of complaining about a problem, find ways to develop a solution. It can be as simple as creating a Power Point presentation to educate others or creating a spreadsheet in Excel that helps your boss to track qualifications and certifications. Regardless of the problem, be tenacious in your pursuit of a solution. Your team will appreciate you and learn to count on you, rather than despise you and dread having to work with you.

Study up and read the latest literature on topics that you encounter most often.

The routine things such as airway management and ventilator maintenance should be at the front of your mind and second-nature. Also as an example , there are many studies regarding IV fluids and choosing the right vasopressor for a particular situation. Read, read, read—then talk to your medical director in the event you think your team needs to make changes in its protocols.

Develop Power Point presentations on topics that you can share with and improve the continuum of care within your community, beginning with firefighters, medics, and staff nurses.

Attend such meetings and conferences as Trauma Mortality and Morbidity at the trauma center that you usually use as your destination. Listen for ways that prehospital care can be improved, ask questions, take notes, and educate your team and referring agencies using your findings. The patients are why we do what we do and anything we can do to improve outcomes is worthy of our time.

Adopt a fire department or ER and devote your time to their training.

Example: Crystal Springs Fire Station in Mississippi. Even considering all of the cool procedures performed and medical decisions made during my nearly 14 years of flying, my favorite times were spent with Crystal Springs Fire and the associated volunteer fire departments—the best days of my career. They were such a super-nice group of go-getters, hungry to learn, and always seemed to enjoy training. Another event you can consider for flight nurses on your team is observing an extrication class in which hydraulic cutting-tools are used. Nurses don't get exposure to that in school and they need to know how to safely operate around that equipment. Plus, you can build great relationships while learning from those agencies you serve.

Social media can help or hurt you.

Be careful to post things that will benefit your team's image. Post pictures of public relations or training events. Don't post pictures of your teammates playing video games with Chinese food boxes adorning tops of desks. Think of social media as your program's advertisement.

Make time to see family members before transport.

It could be easy to get caught up in your assessment, treatment, and packaging for transport, but there's always one more important habit that a FTM should get into: meeting and speaking to the family members of the patient you're transporting. Imagine taking a parent, sibling, or child to the emergency department and then learning that they're being "flown out ". People associate medical helicopters with a bad condition. As you can imagine, that family is experiencing a lot of anxiety. The one thing that you can do to help allay their fears is to briefly stop on your way to the aircraft and talk to them. Introduce yourself and your partner and tell them who you work for and where you're going. Very briefly explain the diagnosis and what you're doing about it (without using medical jargon). After all, we don't just treat patients—we treat their families too.

Follow-up with family members.

This is probably the most important thing you can do after your flights. I always looked at it like they were my family. Would I want my family worrying and wondering what happened to a loved one after they were flown from a crash scene or referring hospital? No. I have never had anyone tell me that they didn't want to hear it. Families of patients were always very appreciative of my taking time to talk with them and answer any questions.

Summary:

Being an effective FTM requires you to be a professional and also a good builder-of-relationships. In closing, I wish you many years of safe flying and the pleasure of being a part of the greatest career in medicine.

CHAPTER 4: PROMOTING A CULTURE

Having a program with an excellent safety record doesn't just happen by accident or automatically. A team has to work at fostering a culture of safety in order to have one. We all want to safely perform our duties at work and return home to our families each day. In order for that goal to be met, as medical crew, there are a few things that we can do to contribute to that cause. Developing a routine, organizing a

team safety committee, and promoting communication among the pilot and medical crews are a great place to start.

Develop a Routine

This aspect of promoting a safety culture by developing a routine includes your inspection of the aircraft and surrounding area while the aircraft is parked at your base. All helipads are set up a little different, so, there's no way to develop a "one-size-fits-all" solution for a routine. This

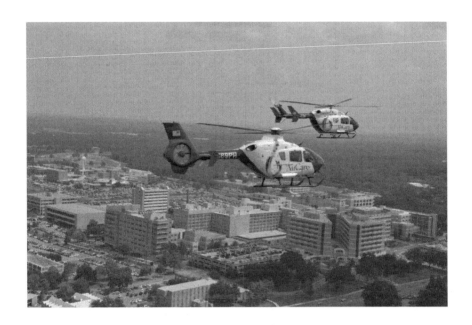

inspection-routine should be used at the beginning of your shift and after you've restocked equipment after your flights. Now, don't think you're going to be opening engine compartments and checking the oil level. For one thing, your pilot will have a coronary event. At this time, I'm talking about identifying issues that are grossly apparent and could result in a less-than-desirable outcome. You should be assuring such things as the shore power being plugged into the aircraft in order to maintain a full charge on your electronic gear. Also, is there any loose debris or dropped medical equipment in the area surrounding the aircraft? I imagine a package of 4x4 gauze or an endotracheal tube blown by rotor wash and sucked up in an engine intake would not be good and may result in someone doing an unseemly amount of paperwork.

In addition, you could look at the aircraft to rule out unfastened latches on compartment access doors, etc. Don't make corrections to the aircraft yourself. Instead, notify the pilot-on-duty and let him/her correct it. Leave the aircraft stuff to your pilot or mechanic. Think about it: would you want your pilot correcting a problem with your defibrillator?

Organize a Team Safety Committee

There are several different ways in which a safety committee can be formed in regards to "who" is on the committee. I can tell you how my team did it and it worked well for us. We had a representative from each discipline on our safety committee. We had a pilot, mechanic, nurse, and a paramedic that could each provide a different perspective on safety issues. Our safety committee would meet for an hour each month, before our regular staff meetings. Any issues brought up in the safety committee meetings would then be passed on in the regular staff meetings, so that everyone was up-to-date on current issues.

Communication Among Pilot and Medical Crew

The worst thing that could happen within a team is to have communication between members, stifled. If "crop-duster, our altitude, about two miles, 9 O'Clock" is replaced by silence because a pilot and a medical crew member aren't getting along, a terrible tragedy could result. Pathways of communication between all team members should remain free-flowing and unimpeded by silly squabbles. Remember, it's your lives we're talking about here.

CHAPTER 5: IFR VS VFR FROM A MEDICAL CREW'S PERSPECTIVE

When I first started flying in July of 1999, our aircraft was an A-Star. It was single-patient capable and limited to flying visual flight rules (VFR). Almost 2 years later, in April 2001, our program invested in an instrument flight rule (IFR)-capable Bell 230. Man, was that 230 cool! It could fly in marginal weather, could accommodate two patients, and had retractable landing gear. It was like flying in the medical version of Airwolf.

How is IFR Different?

From a medical crew's Perspective, the first difference I noticed was that it took us a few extra minutes longer to launch on a flight. Three of the reasons for this are (1) the pilot has to file a flight plan with the FAA, (2) extra fuel had to be put on, and (3) weather briefing and destination weather forecast must be reviewed. Another difference is

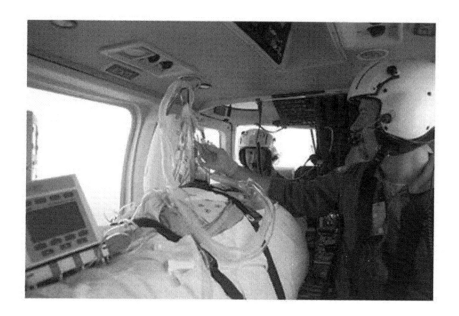

you may not be able to see outside the aircraft due to thick clouds.

What I like about IFR

When flying IFR, I felt the safest. You're always in radio contact and under the control of air traffic control (ATC). ATC helps all IFR-capable aircraft to maintain separation, even when your outside-view is obscured by clouds. The two most striking views during IFR flights is both when you're completely "whited out", or totally enveloped by the clouds, and when you're flying above the cloud tops. It's beautiful up there! The weather on the ground can be foggy, drizzling rain, and dreary, but when you get up above the clouds, it's just a beautiful day. The clouds appear to be an endless white carpet. The other thing I liked about being an IFR program, was that when I was either in or above the clouds, I knew our competition was grounded, since we were the only IFR program in the state. I had a lot of pride in knowing we were still up and doing our thing while everyone else was grounded. I would always gladly take up their slack.

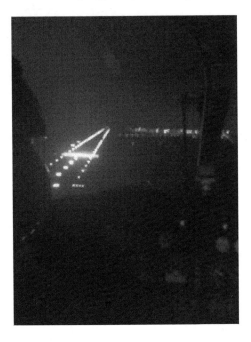

One thing to consider when flying in IFR conditions, is that the instruments may only get you to the airport closest to a patient. Coordination is the name of the game during these flights. You will depend heavily on your communication specialists to assist you with the coordination. You may need an ambulance to meet you at an airport to transport you and your gear to the hospital that the patient is located in. At other times, the ambulance may meet you at the airport with the patient inside. This last scenario was helpful for trauma victims, since minimizing the time it takes to arrive at our level I trauma center greatly improved outcomes.

If you're lucky enough to fly in an IFR program, just remember, planning ahead is a must.

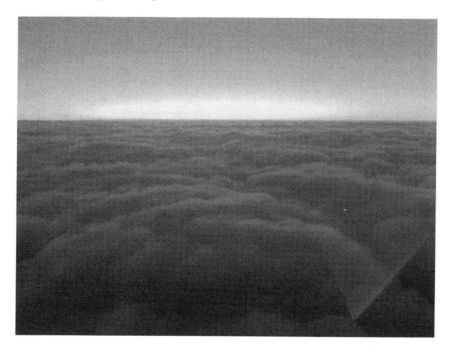

CHAPTER 6: CHECKING YOUR GEAR

In the world of flight medicine, there are two types of medical crew (MC) members: (1) those who check their gear at the beginning of their shift and (2) those who do not. Let me tell you, if you're one of those who do not, your team knows who you are and they don't speak favorably of you. It is important to check your gear for two reasons: (1) you know you have it and (2) you know where it is. The most apparent evidence that you don't appreciate the flying job you have or that your team cannot depend on you, is whether or not you check your gear at the beginning of your shift. For example, to know all of your laryngoscope bulbs work or that you can put your hands on your crico-thyrotomy kit can make the difference between a great shift and an unmitigated disaster. Nothing is worse than needing something and not having it—and you have no one to blame but yourself—except if you walk in the door to a flight, and then it becomes important whether or not the crew before you checked all of the gear. See where I'm going with this? If anyone fails to perform this vital task, the whole team can be negatively impacted.

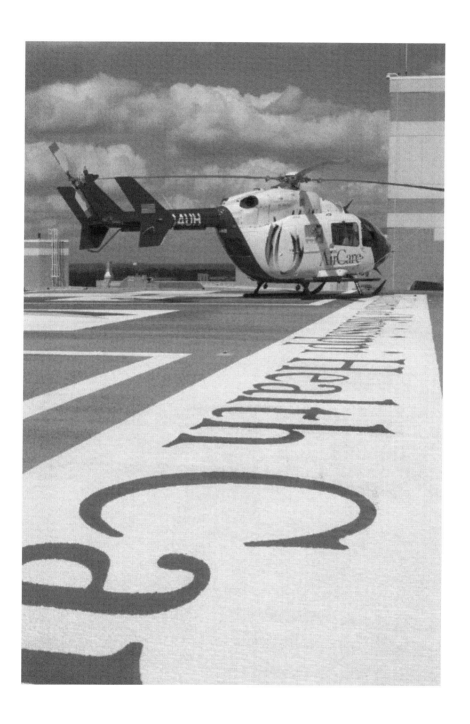

The best way to do this consistently, is to have a standardized list per aircraft, that MC members use each shift. The list of gear should include its location. Checking your gear is the foundation on which you will perform that particular shift. If you start off with a poor foundation, your performance will also be poor. In short, don't be "that" MC member that lets their team and the community they serve, down. Shoot for preparedness and consistency; your shifts will be more productive and effective.

.

CHAPTER 7: COMMUNICATION CENTERS: THE BACKBONE OF ANY FLIGHT TEAM

Flight teams do not function in a vacuum, free of the need for coordination or information. Thankfully, we're fortunate enough to have communication specialists that facilitate a flight team's operation.

I really came to appreciate our communication specialists when we added our second aircraft. The tough decisions they make and the level of coordination they can provide is invaluable. One thing is certain, as flight team members, we couldn't do what we do, if the communication specialists didn't do what they do. One minute they may be taking information for a flight request, the next minute, they're triaging multiple requests, or deciding which aircraft is going to respond to a particular location. Their jobs aren't easy—their's is different from the medical crew's—but every bit as necessary. As medical crew, I don't think we realize how often we call them needing more information or how often we need them to relay an important message to the referring agencies. I was lucky. All of our communication specialists were hard-working people that expected just as much out of themselves as we expected out of ourselves. They "got it " and loved to hear "good job" as much as the medical crew did. Do yourself a favor, show and tell your communication specialists how much you appreciate them. The bottom line is that, considering all of the various moving parts within flight medicine, your communication specialists are the folks that can make your team look great.

CHAPTER 8: SHOOTING FOR GOLDEN CHILD STATUS

You know every team has one. One of those people that are always on time, one that has the shiniest boots, or the one that learns as much as he or she can about the flight medicine business and is always helping the boss with as many projects as possible. At our base in Jackson, MS, we called that kind of person the "Golden Child". I know because I worked really hard for that title!

Look at it like this: your boss has enormous responsibilities and every team can have a slacker or two. Some will hopefully choose to make up for the deficits of others or your boss is going to work him-/herself to death. Again, I was lucky enough to have the greatest boss in the world, Donna Norris. As a flight team member, you likely will not have to worry about the business-end of things. But you can ask what administrative-like projects you can help with. Some examples are: (1) create spreadsheets for tracking certain data or statistics, (2) take charge of re-ordering supplies, or (3) come up with a creative way to track the plethora of qualifications and certifications that are usually maintained by excellent flight teams. I very much respected Donna and I worked very hard to make her life, as manager, as easy as I could.

Tracking Data

One thing you will learn after you start flying is that a tremendous amount of data must be tracked by any flight team. In some cases, the data may be used to change policies and procedures. I think we tracked launch-times for over a year. In the beginning, when we had a trauma flight, we had to pick up two units of O negative blood and we had to go to our medical center's blood bank to pick it up. We found that it caused an unnecessary delay in responding to patients' "golden hour". Using that data, we were able to convince our administrators to provide us with a special refrigerator to store our blood. After that, when we were requested for a flight, we'd simply grab the two units, already in a collapsible cooler, while on the way to the helipad. In this case, tracking data helped our team to be much more efficient.

Reordering supplies

One part of your operation will be reordering and maintaining medical supplies (i.e. IV fluids, syringes, tape, etc.). There must be an organized approach to this duty.

Your team will depend on you to have supplies available when needed and you don't want to let down a team of type-A personalities—you'll lose your golden child status!

Tracking Qualifications/Certifications

In order to be flight medicine material, you should be held to a very high standard in regards to continuing education and maintaining qualifications (i.e. ACLS, PALS, etc.) and certifications (i.e. CEN, CCRN, CFRN, etc.). Tracking currency and expiration dates can be an incredible undertaking for your boss. I would always rather that my boss had free time to ponder my next raise and didn't want her dealing with a task that I felt I was capable of handling. I created this super Excel spreadsheet that I could enter the team members' name, the qualification/certification being tracked, and its expiration date. My boss loved it. I used to take a lot of pride in hearing her describe my projects. She'd say, "Dan not only did it with flash bangs, he'd make it hit you in the head with a 2x4". And you know, as hard as others would try, no one ever came close to stealing my Golden Child Status. Once I retired, everyone else had their chance.

There's nothing more fun than friendly competition among the team. When you have several people trying to outdo one another, in my opinion, you end up with a strong team that you can count on. It is my hope that you learn what it is to be the "Golden Child".

CHAPTER 9: UNFORESEEN REWARDS OF FLIGHT MEDICINE

When one considers a career, usually one considers such things as how much enjoyment can be had, how much would I have to work, or how much money will I make. I will go ahead and tell you that the rewards of flight medicine are so much more than that.

Have you ever been in a tough situation and knew you were meant to be there? As if you were put there or led there to make a difference in somebody's life? Well, I'm going to share two such cases that I will always remember—forever.

We were launched one morning around 10:00 a.m. to a hospital in North Mississippi. It was for a 2-year old with decreased level of consciousness. It was a 50-minute flight and let me tell you that a lot can change in 50 minutes when you're talking about a critically ill child. Well, in this case,

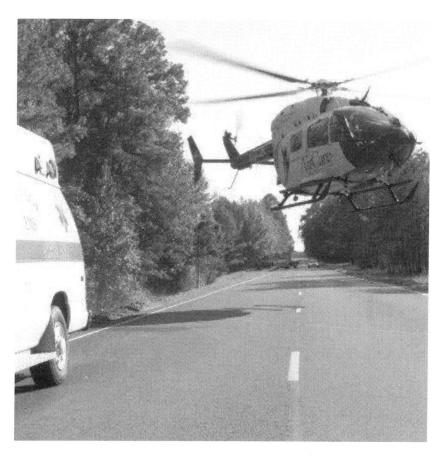

there was a change. Our communication center, MedCom, contacted us on the radio when we were about ten minutes from landing at the referring hospital and said that the child had deteriorated to cardiopulmonary arrest. That's never good to hear. Anyway, we continued on and planned to assist with the resuscitation. We landed and was met by a friendly security guard that had a stretcher for our gear and he escorted my partner and me to the patient's room. A respiratory therapist met us outside the patient's door and told us that the doctor had just pronounced the patient dead. I could hear several people crying inside the room. In this situation, there's nothing we can do, but I felt like there was something that I could offer—comfort to a family that I didn't even know. You know how uncomfortable it can be comforting someone you know who has lost a loved-one. Imagine how difficult it could be trying to comfort someone you don't know. I couldn't help it. Hearing their sorrowful cries just broke my heart and I couldn't leave without trying. My partner at the time was a flight paramedic, named Casey Campbell. Casey is a very intelligent guy with one of the best personalities anyone could ask for—everybody loved Casey. Anyway, instead of packing our gear and leaving, I mentioned to Casey, "Let's go in and talk to them". So, Casey and I walked into the room and introduced ourselves and told them we were with the flight team from UMMC. I asked them what was their little boy's name and what happened. There were four or five family members standing in a circle around the bed where the dead child laid. Knowing that we couldn't stay forever, I asked everyone if they'd be offended if I said a prayer before we left. I heard an emphatic, "Please do"! We all joined hands and aloud, I prayed that God would see him safely to Heaven and prayed for His comfort and strength during this extremely difficult time. When I finished, two of the family members also wanted to say a prayer. It was a very cool and unforgettable moment during my career. After the last prayer was said, Casey and I said our "goodbyes", gathered our gear, loaded up, and lifted off to return to our base at UMMC. On the way home, Casey said something to me that meant a lot and I never forgot what kind of impact I could have on people without ever touching a syringe, medication, or any other gear. Casey said, "Dan, you are truly a healer". That meant so much to me and I was honored to have helped provide comfort during a family's worst day. That day very much shaped me into a better flight nurse. Thank you, Casey Campbell.

A second case in which I felt that I was led to a tragedy for a reason other than our state-of-the-art equipment and extensive training was at the scene of a car wreck for a teenager. This is another one of those cases when you only think you know why you're flying to help someone. However ,you end up touching more lives than you were launched for. There was a head-on collision with a high schooler trapped inside with lower extremity deformities. Once we landed, I performed a quick primary survey to make sure we had an adequate airway, breathing, and circulation. All were acceptable and I assured the patient, Colby, that I'd take good care of him and I would give him some medicine to help with his pain. After making contact with Colby, I got out of the firemen's way so they could complete the use of their hydraulic tools and I noticed what seemed to be Colby's parents. They were watching intently and had such a look of anguish on their faces. I walked over to introduce myself and to let them know that I'd be taking good care of their son. I swear I felt their spirits ease as we talked. Colby's parents are Mark and Anita Rigdon. Below is written correspondence from Anita and Mark. It describes their perspective of the extrication, treatment, transport, and follow-up in the days to come:

Letter from Anita Rigdon

"February 8, 2012, is a day that I will never forget. Our son Colby was in a head on collision and he was trapped in the car. As we watched the emergency responders trying to get him out I remember hearing a helicopter and seeing it circling over us. I asked "what in the world is going on", and one of the emergency responders told me that they were looking for a place to land so they could take Colby to the hospital from the scene. What seemed like moments later, a young man by the name of Dan Turner introduced himself to Mark and I and said he would be taking care of Colby once they got him out of the car. He told us from what he could see he thought he could just be transported to Meridian but once they got Colby out he looked at us and said "we are headed to UMC" and assured us he would take care of him. When we got to the hospital we did not see the Air-flight team. However, Dan found us! He told us of how on the flight over Colby had been so calm and had led them in prayer and what an impression Colby had made on him. Colby had 2 broken legs and was in fear of loosing one of his feet. Dan prayed and cried with us that day in the hospital room and made a lasting impression on us all. Colby told him of his desire to work in the medical field and Dan offered to help him in anyway he could. Dan and the UMC Air-flight team are wonderful, caring people. I see, from time to time, the UMC helicopter come over our house and I am always reminded of how one day we needed that helicopter and those special people on board."

Letter from Mark Rigdon

"I met Dan about 8:30am on Wednesday February 8th 2012, near Union MS. My son, Colby, had been involved in a head-on collision on his way to school. This was the last semester of his senior year. We got to the scene about 15 minutes after it happened and had been watching our local fire department trying to cut him out of the car. About the time we saw the helicopter, the fire chief came and told us the team on board were landing to take Colby to the hospital. When the helicopter landed we met Dan. He let us know he was going to take care of Colby and I think Dan's demeanor and confidence brought calm to me. This was my first dealings with any sort of emergency rescue and transport. I can't describe it but the connection with Dan was instant. In the days to follow, Dan and his partner visited us and Dan told us about Colby praying with him during the flight and how Colby made an impression on him . I can tell you that there were no dry eyes in that hospital room that day!

The overall impression of Dan and his team was great. I think about that day every time I see an Air Care helicopter fly over the house and that someone is in trouble and there is a GREAT team up there helping.

In the nearly 6 years that have passed, Colby Rigdon has done some incredible things. He was accepted into an ADN program out of high school and became a RN in 2 years—

then worked and upgraded to a BSN degree over the next year. All of this between about 8 surgeries on his right foot. He is currently working at River Oaks in the ER and part time in the Cath Lab at Merit Central. You would be as proud as I am!"

Let me tell you, to get that kind of feedback is better than any payday you can receive. In my career, I had no greater responsibility than that of taking care of peoples' sons and daughters. It was an honor and privilege to have had that role. Thanks a million to Mark and Anita for their kind words. Flight medicine isn't just measured by how well you perform procedures or how many successful resuscitations you've had. It's also measured by your ability to be the best part of someone's worst day. Many times, in addition to our medical expertise, we simply need to treat others as if they're our family. I always lived by the "mama rule". If you treat everyone like you'd want your mama to be treated, you will never, ever go wrong.

CHAPTER 10: THE FINAL CHAPTER

This one is the hardest chapter to write. Throughout this book I have relived happy and proud moments. This one reminds me that it all had to end—way too soon. I guess I should try to judge whether or not I ever achieved excellence. I know that I worked very hard in my pursuit of excellence. I lived, ate, drank, and breathed flight medicine. I put my all into my career. Do I have any regrets? Yes—I regret leaving the house on my Harley that fateful day, December 8, 2012. But, I have no regrets as to my career choice or how I tried to represent my team. I strived every day to be what I thought a flight team member should be. I made some lifelong friendships during some pretty difficult times. Whether it was in a referring hospital's ER or upside down in a rolled over vehicle, I gave it my all. So, in that

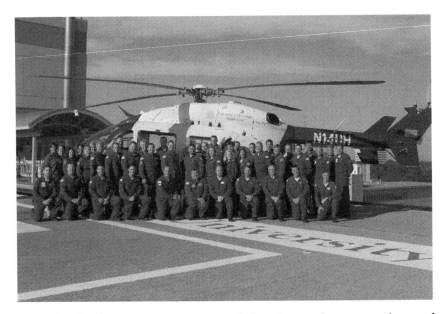

regard, I had a great career—and thanks to the examples and people who helped shape my career, I successfully pursued and achieved excellence.

ABOUT THE AUTHOR

This book was written by a flight team member of University of Mississippi Medical Center's AirCare helicopter critical care transport team.. This book is meant to provide a comprehensive guide to flight medicine for registered nurses and paramedics who are interested in a career in flight medicine, as well as, laypeople who are simply curious about the greatest career one can have in medicine.

My name is Dan Turner and I am very proud to have been a flight nurse for 13 1/2 years at University of Mississippi Medical Center's AirCare. I was forced to retire at age 40, disabled, after sustaining a traumatic brain injury that resulted from hitting a deer while riding my Harley. The upper motor neurons of my brainstem were injured, leaving me with left-sided weakness. Cognitively, I have no issues. However, physically, I do. One thing I regret most is not being able to fly anymore. I have always wanted to share with the world, what I learned during the best years of my life. When I first began to consider flight medicine as a career, there was not one book that explained, comprehensively, what flight medicine was about. It is my hope that this book will serve as such a reference.

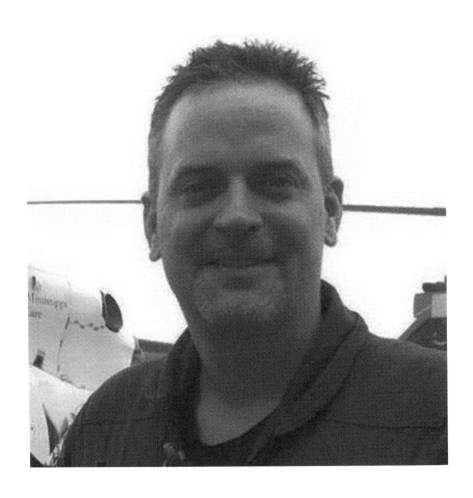

Made in the USA
Columbia, SC
30 January 2019